Yoga

Your Ultimate Beginner's Guide On How To Use Yoga To Maximize Weight Loss And Live The Stress-Free Life Of Your Dreams!

Table of Contents

Introduction

I want to thank you and congratulate you for buying the book "Yoga: Your Ultimate Beginner's Guide On How To Use Yoga To Maximize Weight Loss And Live The Stress-Free Life Of Your Dreams!"

This book contains proven steps and strategies on how to incorporate yoga into your daily routine and get the best of it.

Many people have a completely skewed image of what yoga really is. Don't trust what others say. Make the effort and find out for yourself what it is. Discover what yoga really represents and how it can help you transform your life into a life really worth living.

Thanks again for buying this book, I hope you enjoy it!

Chapter 1: What Is Yoga?

Finding yourself on the threshold of this new and exciting journey, you will certainly be asking yourself this question: what is yoga really? The answer to this is as simple (or as complicated) as you yourself want it to be. Different people use it for different purposes, all highly effective ones. But, in essence, the word yoga is the Sanskrit word for add, join, unite, and thus, in its noun form, it means unity or connection. It is an ancient art that re-establishes the connection between your body, mind, and soul. It is a journey that will lead you to peace and well-being.

In today's fast-paced life, we are looking for easy solutions to solve our problems, and so we tend to look for sources of fulfillment and gratification outside ourselves. This is the age of instant gratification; we are thirsty for easy, simple, and quick solutions. And, we search for the answers to our queries everywhere else but within us. We are all too eager busy focusing on the materialistic side of life, neglecting (either consciously or subconsciously) the spiritual side. But, as some of the well-known teachers will tell you, you cannot be truly happy if the source of your happiness is external. Your joy, your enthusiasm, and motivation should come from within you. For example, if your profession is something that was chosen for you, or that you chose simply based on the paycheck you would be getting, it is quite possible that this kind of job doesn't bring you too much pleasure. On the contrary, when you are doing a job that fulfils you, which you chose based on your own inner motivations, you will find yourself beaming with satisfaction and joy.

So, if you are looking forward to a journey that would bring you happiness from within, then you are in the right place. Yoga is a (seemingly) simplistic practice of directing this flow of energy inwards. Through this practice you will be able to introspect and enjoy a stress-free state of mind, deriving pleasure that doesn't come from any outside sources, but rather from your own contentment with your own life.

You will be able to establish harmony with your own True Self, an ego-free happy self. You become one with your own thoughts and accept yourself for who you are, without boasting about your virtues and despising your vices. You will become the true you, and as such a worthy individual whose thoughts matter. Yoga, when incorporated as a quintessential element of your life, could help you achieve this state of mind, at the same time empowering you to change, surrender and let go of all other aspects of your life that do not serve you physically, emotionally, or spiritually.

To put it simply, yoga could help you center your energy and bring you peace of mind, enhanced self-esteem and self-confidence. In addition, it helps you stay healthy, fit, and in shape, while improving your balance, posture and flexibility, eliminating tension and pain from your muscles, and much more.

At its very heart, yoga is for every single person. Whether you are trying to create a new healthier lifestyle by controlling your food intake, reducing your stress levels or focusing more intently on solving your problems without anxiety, yoga can definitely be the right choice for you.

Yoga is like a bouquet filled with lusciously fragrant flowers, from which you are allowed to pick the one you need. But, today, this form of art has become synonymous with an exercise regimen that would help you shed the excess flab and de-stress your life. While these benefits do exist, as aforementioned, there is much more yoga can give you.

And, that is why you all are here today, reading this book. Welcome to the world of Yoga. Begin your journey today with this book as your guide into a life filled with pure happiness, joy and wellness!

Along with three simple routines that will help you rid yourself of the excess weight and stress, this book also provides you with everything you need to know about yoga. From the various myths about yoga to all you'll ever need for a home-based practice, from simple tips to some essential poses aimed at enhancing your life, this book offers it all.

So are you ready for this journey?

Fasten your seatbelts and gear up for an interesting Yoga journey with me!

Chapter 2: Basic Misconceptions About Yoga

Can you remember how many times you've shared your idea about taking up yoga, only to be met with surprised, staring looks from those around you? And then, dead silence, because, hey, what is there to say to that? Whoever gave you that awfully uncomfortable look a few years ago (which by the way, made you stop thinking about yoga for a while) is not the only one who thinks this way. But, don't worry. Just because a lot of people think this way, it still doesn't make their opinions true or factual. Here are a few basic misconceptions which people generally tend to have when it comes to yoga.

Yoga is a girly practice (and no real man would ever do it!)

While it is true that you'd mostly see women at yoga practice, it is also true that some of the masters of yoga are men (surprise, surprise!). The same goes for chefs, too. But, back to yoga. Men are generally used to high frequency work outs, burning calories like crazy and basically not leaving the gym other than to work, sleep and eat. Not that we're saying this is bad. But, men can get in great shape through yoga, too, especially since there are numerous new combinations of power yoga, Ashtanga yoga and many others. So, leave your prejudices at the door, and ask yourself: Are you man enough for yoga?

It's all stretching and no real work

Boy, this could not be further from the truth. In the beginning, it might appear that most of the things you do are easy and ineffective, but just you wait. The practice affects you immediately, and as you advance to higher levels (eventually being able to twist yourself into a pretzel!), you'll see how much hard work it is trying to stay in these complicated poses for more than a couple of seconds.

You have to be X to practice yoga

Many people tend to think that you have to be one of the following things to practice yoga: thin, strong, flexible, young-ish. Wrong. Why else do you think it's called yoga practice? Practice implies you start with the simple version of something, and in time, you become as good as you want to be. It's as easy as that. Just remember that practice makes perfect and go to that first yoga class!

It's a religion (and I already have mine)

Even though yoga is a spiritual practice, it is not religion. It is not a different name for Buddhism or Hinduism, it's just that these religions chose to incorporate this practice into their spiritual development. You can belong to any religion you want and practice yoga without fear of religious retribution from your priest.

If you practice yoga, you will become X

X in this case stands for vegetarian, vegan, hippie, minimalist, you name it. You don't have to change any of the habits you love because of yoga. Yoga changes only those habits that are preventing you from reaching spiritual balance.

Yoga is dangerous

While some think yoga exercises are too easy, there is the other extreme of people thinking it's too hard and it's bound to be dangerous. As it was already mentioned, it's a practice, so of course your yoga teacher won't allow you to try advanced exercises without having mastered the initial ones.

Hopefully, we've managed to eradicate these misconceptions from your mind, and you can now see and accept the fact that yoga isn't the boogeyman of physical exercise.

Chapter 3: Benefits Of Yoga

Yoga has numerous benefits for your physical as well as psychological state of mind. In the following few lines, we tried to break it down to the best of the best.

Physical benefits

- **Improved flexibility**

One of the initial changes in your body that you will witness (to your joy). You might not be able to reach your toes during the first week, but don't give up. The more you practice, the more flexible your muscles and joints will become, allowing your limbs and spine to bend beyond the point you ever thought possible.

- **Improved posture**

Don't you just love how graceful ballerinas are? How they don't move, but rather flow through the air? Well, you can become like them with yoga. Granted, you might not be able to skip so gracefully and do a pirouette, but you will have the posture of a royal ballerina, with an elongated spine, shoulders back and neck straightened.

- **Muscle strength**

No one wants to look flabby. And in order not to look flabby, you have to tighten your muscles. Yoga poses do exactly that: they keep your body and muscles tight for a certain period of time, building core muscle and prolonging the effect.

- **Improved blood circulation**

Truth be told, any kind of physical exercises gets your heart pumping and your blood boiling. However, yoga has the added benefits of flowing your blood from your legs back towards your heart, through poses like the headstand, the handstand and the shoulder stand, which reduce the risk of varicose veins.

- **Reduced tension in your limbs**

We all have these subconscious habits we aren't aware of. Sometimes it's the tight grip of the steering wheel, at others it's the fact that we spend a lot of time on our phones, keeping our arms bent in an uncomfortable position. This all takes its toll on the muscles, which then become tight (but, not the good kind of tight), and it's difficult to relax them. Yoga can help you with this. Breathing exercises, along with effective poses can target the tension in your muscles and alleviate it.

- **Boosting the immune system**

Interestingly enough, studies have shown that yoga can help you raise the level of antibodies when necessary, which is very important during flu seasons. So, instead of taking vitamin pills to boost your immunity, opt for more fruits and veggies in combination with yoga. You'll be amazed with the results!

- **Pain reduction**

Other studies have proved that certain aspects of yoga, such as meditation and asana (the poses), can be very beneficial in treating people with chronic conditions, like arthritis, fibromyalgia and back pain. As it relieves pain, yoga helps you focus on being more active, targeting pain areas and lowering the soreness.

Psychological benefits

- **Relaxation**

The first thing you might feel after your initial yoga class is how relaxed you are. Well, get ready for feeling better and better every time you do yoga, because as you teach your mind to relax and let go of all that bothers it, you will be able to find a peace of mind, and this will in turn, make your life much more beautiful. Because, when we're under stress, we tend to neglect the beauty of every day details. Once you've uncluttered your mind, the world will seem like a much brighter place.

- **Improved ability to focus**

While we hate to admit it, it is true: we so often tend to live in the past, reliving our mistakes and wrong choices, instead of focusing on the present, trying to find out how to fix those mistakes in the past and learn from them, and enjoy the present. Carpe Diem, right? Well, luckily for you, yoga can help there, too. It urges you to focus on the present, on what you are doing right now, not what you were doing or will do. Now is the time to take action.

- **Improved sleeping pattern**

Once you allow yoga to wake you up spiritually, you can allow it to lull you back to sleep as well. Of course it's a great thing to be stimulated, but the body as well as the mind needs to rest properly. How many times did you catch yourself counting sheep, only to reach an insane number and find out it's already time to go to work? Well, that's not good. Lack of sleep affects both your mood and your performance, so if you didn't rest well, chances are you won't be leaving a good impression on your boss the following day. Who knows, lack of sleep might even cost you a promotion! Don't let this happen. Yoga provides stress release through meditation and relaxing poses. This way, you are able to zone out and provide some much needed rest for your system.

- **Greater self-esteem**

Most parents teach their children to be modest. And, it's a good thing to be. But sometimes, it happens that modesty transforms into chronic lack of self-esteem. This affects every area of our lives: we might miss out on a good job opportunity (because we didn't leave a good impression, thinking ourselves not worthy of the position) or even on meeting a prospective life partner (as people with low self-esteem don't have the courage to approach the people they find attractive). Furthermore, people who suffer from lack of self-esteem, tend to compensate for this in very negative ways, like overeating, oversleeping, transforming into a workaholic, even indulging excessively in drugs and alcohol. Needless to say, these lead nowhere, simply because the problem isn't outside. The problem is within us. The introspective approach to yoga can help people with low self-esteem re-examine their own lives and the choices that led them there. Then, the focus turns to betterment and continual self-examination for the purpose of achieving something bigger, something better: a happy you.

- **Greater inner strength**

This aspect is closely connected with self-esteem. The more self-confident we are, the more eager we are to take our lives into our own hands and create something magical out of it. We tend to eradicate our dysfunctional habits, substitute them with positive ones and continually endeavor to live in the moment, seize the day and never miss out on something that could potentially be the best choice we have ever made.

- **Creating a basis for a healthier lifestyle**

Like any other kind of physical exercise, yoga helps keep your mind and body happy and healthy. You burn calories, you stress less, you focus and concentrate more, and surprise, surprise, you might also realize that fast food is bad for you. While no one will judge you for indulging in an occasional hamburger, French fries or cheesecake, you might realize yourself that overdoing this isn't such a good idea and that you can always make healthier, and equally yummy versions of this food at home, turning you into a mindful eater.

- **Bettering your relationships**

Whether you are the kind of person who shies from expressing his or her emotions freely, or the kind of person who hugs everyone, there are always meaningful ways to show someone how much you appreciate them. Practicing yoga helps you keep calm and happy, which in turns allows you to feel greater compassion, friendliness and love for those around you. The spiritual side of yoga teaches you to avoid hurting others, both people and animals, to appreciate others and be grateful, to avoid telling lies and expressing your honest opinion. This can prove to be invaluable in your social interactions.

Chapter 4: Different Types Of Yoga

Like any other physical activity and sport, yoga also offers several different versions, and we're sure you'll be able to find the one most suited to you.

1. Hatha Yoga

Hatha yoga is what most people are familiar with. It consists mostly of basic yoga postures anyone can do, making it perfect for a beginner. What's best about it is that it won't make you sweat much, but you'll still have your work out, and you will leave your yoga studio feeling as if your body has somehow become more elongated, as well as more relaxed.

2. Vinyasa Yoga

The Sanskrit word meaning "flow," vinyasa yoga is slightly more intense than hatha yoga, and it is similar to ashtanga yoga. There is a smoother transition from one pose to another, and there is usually calming music playing in the background, inducing a greater sense of relaxation. It aims to test one's physical limits, and keep things out of the rut.

3. Ashtanga Yoga

Similar to vinyasa, though ashtanga tends to focus on a routine, and in class, you will mostly repeat the same poses in the same order. However, don't doubt its impact: you'll be cringing inside, as this is one seriously sweaty workout.

4. Anusara Yoga

Anusara yoga focuses on intrinsic goodness, combining the physical side of yoga with the person's own inner light. If you're looking for something that will bring about not only a relaxation and a peace of mind, but a unification of the body and the soul, then look no further. This is your ticket.

5. Bikram Yoga

Bikram yoga consists of 26 poses, and it is widely popular among yogis. It also focuses on sequence which never changes (though it differs from ashtanga). What's interesting here is that you'll work out a double sweat, seeing that this yoga session is held in a heated room.

6. Restorative Yoga

You might be looking for a way to restore some of your nerves (because, let's face it, we only have so many of them), and restorative yoga offers passive poses which will help you with exactly this. Its main goal is to rejuvenate you and make you feel better and more charged up than if you had a nap or an energy drink.

7. Yin Yoga

It is generally considered a type of restorative yoga, but it is ideally a great way to balance the Yang or the most strenuous yoga types which we generally practice. The focus is on rejuvenating the connective tissues, which in turn will help open up the tough zones in your body, making you more flexible.

Chapter 5: Essential Equipment

While there's no crucial mistake that you can make when it comes to preparing for your first ever yoga class, there are a few things worth knowing. Just for your own personal peace of mind. Firstly, you need to wear comfy clothes. Nowadays, the choices are numerous, so choose whatever makes you want to get busy, but make sure to wear form-fitting clothes, due to all the bending and twisting. You don't want to give anyone a show they haven't paid a ticket for, right? As far as shoes as concerned, yoga is best done without any (and without socks).

So, here are a few pieces of equipment you need to get familiar with:

1. Mats.

Also known as a sticky mat and widely used in all yoga classes. You need your personal space while doing poses, so it marks what's yours, plus it helps you when your hands get all sweaty and sticky, because it keeps you from slipping. I'd suggest buying one of your own, as there is a high chance of it not being washed very frequently, which is the case at many yoga studios (just think how many people use it on a daily basis). You can find one for as low as 20$, so if you value your hygiene, it's totally worth it.

2. Towels.

Not that it's a major part of the equipment, but oh so useful. If you don't know whether your yoga studio will provide one for you, make sure to bring one from home.

3. Blankets.

Yoga studios should provide these. You're to use it as a prop basically, while lying or sitting. It's especially useful for beginners.

4. Straps.

If you're still a beginner or you can't clasp your hands or hold onto your feet, straps will come in mighty handy. But don't worry, no one is expecting you to bring them from home.

5. Blocks.

Another supportive instrument which can help you in some poses you still find a bit tricky.

6. Bolsters.

Bolsters come to the rescue when you need to recline in certain poses as well as while practicing certain breathing techniques.

Chapter 6: Basic Moves

No one likes to go somewhere for the first time and not know what to expect. So that you can avoid this uncomfortable situation, here are a few beginner yoga poses that your yoga teacher will introduce you to during your first couple of classes.

- **Accomplished Pose (Siddhasana)**

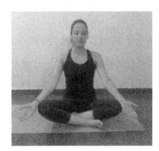 You are in a seated position, and one heel is right between your groin, while the other is on top, with the foot resting on the calf. Your back should be completely straight, arms resting on the knees. This pose is mostly used for meditation and deep breathing.

- **Hero Pose (Virasana)**

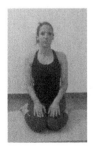 The hero pose is another great pose for meditation and breathing, and it is also a beginning position for many bending and twisting poses. You should be seated, with your calves and feet slightly away from your body, pointing backwards. Your back should be straight, arms resting on your thighs.

- **Thunderbolt Pose/Kneeling (Vajrasana)**

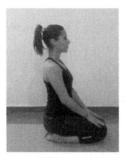

Kneel on the floor, allowing the buttocks to rest on the heels. Keep the knees and feet together. Straighten the spine and lengthen the torso. Let the palms rest on the thighs.

- **Downward-Facing Dog (Adho Mukha Svanasana)**

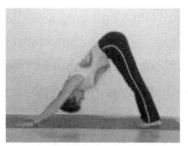

The easiest way to start this pose is being on your hands and knees: hands beneath your shoulders, knees beneath your hips. As you curl your toes, lift your hips and made a downward V with your body. Your chest is pushing towards your knees, eyes on your toes, heels firmly on the floor.

- **Cobra (Bhujangasana)**

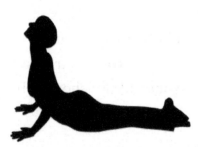

Lie down on the floor, on your stomach, with tops of your feet flat. On an inhale, press the palms and top of the feet into the floor and lift your head, chest, and torso up. Lift your upper body until your navel. Your hips should rest on the floor. Keep the elbows bent. Engage the core, thighs, and buttocks and hold the posture. Exhale and lie down on your stomach.

- **Warrior 1 (Virabhadrasana I)**

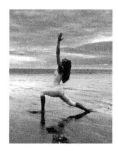

Stand straight with your feet in contact, hands resting along your body. Inhale and place the right leg back, about three feet away from the left foot, turning the right foot towards the right at 45 degrees. Exhale, bend your left knee, stacking it over your left ankle. Allow your left thigh to come parallel to the floor. Inhale and swing your hands over your head, aligning it with your ears. Engage the core, keep the hips squared to the front, and gaze at a point in front of you. Hold the posture, breathing deeply, for a couple of breaths. Inhale and join the feet and relax your hands. Repeat on the other side.

- **Warrior 2 (Virabhadrasana II)**

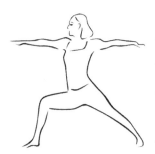

Stand up straight, with arms next to your body, tight. As you inhale, step your left leg back about three feet away from the front foot. Exhale and bend left foot 90 degrees. It should face forward, while the right foot faces slightly to the left side. Bring your left knee is parallel to the floor, keeping your right leg is straight... Spread your arms front and back, keeping them aligned. Gaze at a point in front of you while hips are squared to the left. Inhale and join the feet, Repeat on the other side.

- **Tree Pose (Vriksasana)**

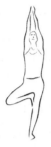

Stand straight. Shift weight to left leg. Bend the right leg at knee and rest the right foot on your left inner thigh. Make sure that the right knee is pointing towards the right. Pull your navel in and join your palms at your chest. Fix your gaze at one point. If you are comfortable here, lift your arms over your head and join your palms. Hold the posture, breathing deeply. On an exhalation, release the right foot and palms. Repeat the same on the other side.

- **Mountain Pose (Tadasana)**

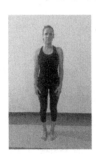

The basic standing position. Stand upright, with feet close together and hands next to the body. Fingers together, stretched downward.

- **Lion Pose (Simhasana)**

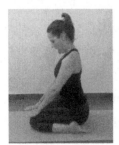

Start by kneeling on the floor, feet pointing outwards, while you are sitting comfortably on the inner tops of your heels. Palms resting on your knees. Fingers outstretched. Take a deep breath, open your mouth as wide as you can and stick your tongue out, stretching it downwards. Eyes wide open. Exhale with a powerful "ha" sound. For additional fun, feel free to roar a few times.

- **Chair pose (Utkatasana)**

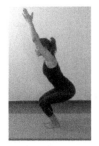

Begin with Mountain Pose. Feet together (beginners - feet slightly apart). Inhale and raise your arms above your head. Exhale and bend your knees. Bring the thighs parallel to the floor as much as possible. Stack your knees over your ankles. Make sure that your toes are visible. Roll back your shoulders and press the feet firmly into the mat. Gaze forward. Engaging the abdominal muscles, breathe deeply.

- **Plank Pose (Dandasana/Khumbakasana)**

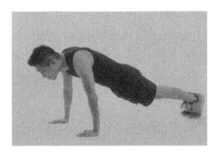

Start with Downward Facing Dog pose. Come on your toes. As you inhale, push your torso forward in such a way that you are stacking your shoulders over your wrists. Spread the fingers wide. Engage your core and align your body in such a way that it looks like a straight line from head to toe. Breathe into the pose to hold it longer.

- **Child's Pose (Balasana)**

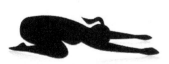

Start from a kneeling position. Let the buttocks rest on your heels. Inhale and swing your arms over your head. Exhale and fold forward, resting your abdomen on the thighs and forehead on the floor. Let your hands rest on either sides of your forehead or make a pillow with your hand and rest your forehead on that. Breathe deeply into the posture to relax better.

- ## Corpse Pose (Savasana)

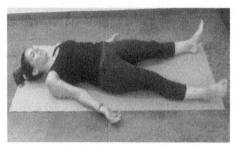

Lie down flat on your back, legs separated wider than your hips, allowing the feet to fall naturally to the sides. Spread your hands away from the body, palms facing the ceiling, fingers curled naturally, giving enough space for your armpits to breath. Tuck your chin slightly towards the chest to relax your neck. Close your eyes and consciously relax your entire body. Breathing normally, relax yourself.

- ## Sun salutation (Surya Namaskara)

It is a gentle Vinyasa sequence which the beginners can practice. There are different variations of Sun Salutations. The one mentioned below is the classical one which comprises 12 poses.

Pranamasana/Samasthithi

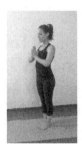

Stand with your feet together. Join your palms at your heart center. Roll back your shoulders, engage the core, thighs, and buttocks. Lengthen the spine. Press the feet firmly into the floor and stretch your neck as if you are pulling your body towards the ceiling. Fix your gaze at the fingertips. Take 3 rounds of deep inhalations and exhalations.

Hasta Uttanasana

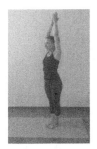

Remaining in the same standing position, lift your hands slowly above your head, keeping them together. Stretch as far as is comfortable. Inhale deeply as you do this.

Hasta padasana/Uttanasana

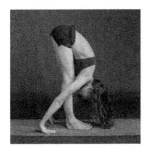

Exhale and fold forward from the hips and place your palms on either sides of your feet, allowing the head to come close to the shin while abdomen rests on the thighs. You can keep the knees gently bent if your palms do not touch the floor or you have a back or knee injury. Keep the core muscles and thighs engaged. Push the hips back and lengthen the spine.

Aekpaadprasarnaasana/Aswa Sanchalanasana

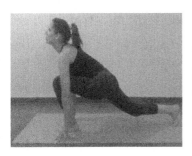

Inhale and place your right leg back as much as possible, balancing yourself on the toes, while bending the left knee and stacking it over the left ankle. Come on your fingertips and lift the chest off the thighs. Gaze forward. Feel free to keep the back knee down, if you find it difficult to hold the posture.

Dandasana (Plank Pose) - Exhale from the previous pose and come into Plank.

Ashtanga Namaskara / Knee – Chest- Chin

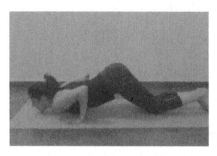 From Dandasana, hold the breath and place your knees on the mat. Place your chest in between your palms and chin on the floor at the same time.

Bhujangasana (Cobra) - Taking an inhalation, scoop your body forward and come into Cobra Pose.

Adho Mukha Svanasana (Downward Facing Dog) – Exhale, tuck your toes, and come into Downward Facing Dog pose.

Aekpaadprasarnaasana - Inhale and place your right foot in between your palms. Keep the right knee bent and stacked over your right ankle, while the left leg remains straight. Feel free to keep the left knee down on the mat, if you are not able to balance.

Hastapaadasana – Exhale and place your left foot next to the right and complete your forward fold.

Hasta Uttanasana – Inhale, sweep your hands over your head and take a gentle backbend.

Pranamasana - Exhale and join your palms at your heart center.

This completes only half of one round of Surya Namaskara. Repeat on the other side to complete one round.

Now that you know some of the basic poses, it shouldn't be so scary going for the first time, right?

Chapter 7: The 7-Minute Weight Loss Sequence

Exercising is one of the quintessential ingredients of a weight loss expedition. However, there are moments when we really don't feel like getting into those tracks and tees and hitting the gym or visiting our yoga classes. And, most of us feel so guilty about this that we end up overeating. It's a vicious cycle to which there is no end.

But do not worry. Here is a solution to break this cycle. You just need 7 minutes to do this sequence and it gives your metabolism a superb high, helping you with your weight loss.

Wait! Wait! There is something more I would like to share with you before you get to know the sequence. While this is a small sequence, you can do it 7 times to create your own one-hour workout schedule as the yoga poses mentioned are pretty simple, yet fabulously effective. Your core, thighs, and arms are targeted in all the poses.

7 Minutes To Fat Burning

The poses should be practiced in the mentioned order without taking any breaks and holding each one for one minute.

Prepare with Samasthithi – The Equilibrium

Start your journey in Samasthithi. Stand straight, with your feet in contact, hands resting on either sides of your body, spine, neck and head aligned. Roll back your shoulders away from the ears. Lengthen your torso as if you are trying to touch the ceiling with your head. Press the feet deep onto the mat/floor. Close your eyes and take three deep inhalations and exhalations, preparing your body and mind for the practice.

1. Chair Pose (Utkatasana)

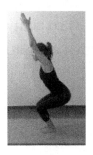 A great way to tone your thighs and abdomen, it helps to promote metabolism and strengthening your spine.

1. With the final exhalation in Samasthithi, bend the knees while pushing the hip back like you are sitting on an imaginary chair.

2. Pull your navel close to the spine and engage the abdominal muscles. Tuck your tailbone in and keep the hips squared.

3. Adjust your knees in such a way that they are right over your ankles and your toes are visible.

4. Straighten your torso in such a way that it makes a 45 degree angle with your thighs.

5. Inhale, sweep your arms over your head and join the palms.

6. Tilt your head back gently and gaze at the fingertips.

7. Hold the posture for one minute, breathing deeply.

2. Revolved Lunge (Parivrtta Parsvakonasana)

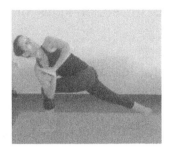

Detoxification is essential to promote weight loss and this posture helps you with that. It also stimulates your digestion and tones your abdomen, hips, and legs.

1. Once you complete Chair Pose, inhale and place your left leg back, at least three feet away from your right foot. Tuck the toes of your left foot. Keep the right knee bent.

2. Exhale and twist from your waist to the right, bringing the joined palms outside the right knee. Open your chest to the right.

3. Sink your hips further down to keep the left leg straight and active. Engage your core and gaze at the ceiling.

4. Hold the posture for one minute, breathing deeply.

Tips: You can place the left knee on the mat if you find this difficult.

3. Plank (Khumbhakasana/Dandasana)

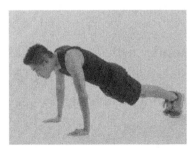

This just sets the heat on. So, beware! If your core is weak, then this pose will set it right with regular practice.

1. Once you complete the previous posture, inhale and untwist your torso. Place your palms on either sides of your right foot.

2. On the next exhalation, place your right leg back, tucking the toes, next to your left ofoot.

3. Adjust your arms so that the wrists are right beneath your shoulders. Spread the fingers out wide.

4. Engage your core and let the legs be active. Squeeze your buttocks.

5. Adjust your hips in such a way that they are neither sinking nor going towards the ceiling. The entire body should be in a single line. [Refer to the image] Balance yourself on the toes.

6. Hold the posture, breathing in and out of the abdomen, for one minute.

Tips: *Place your forearms on the mat to balance your body on the elbows. Lower your body so that it comes parallel to the floor.*

4. Upward Facing Dog Pose (Urdhva Mukha Svanasana)

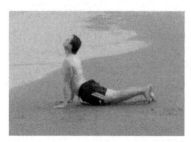

It is a gentle arm balance that works wonderfully towards toning your entire body, including the legs and back.

1. From the Plank, exhale and drop your knees on the floor, allowing the tops of the feet to rest on the mat.

2. Inhale and push the hips forward and down toward the floor.

3. Pressing the palms into the mat, exhale and roll back your shoulders. Simultaneously, push the chest forward and drop your head back to gaze at the ceiling.

4. On an inhale, push the tops of feet firmly into the mat and lift your thighs and knees off the mat, balancing your entire body on the palms and feet. Keep the core, thigh, and butt muscles engaged and active.

5. Taking deep breaths, hold the posture for one minute.

5. Downward Facing Dog Pose (Adho Mukha Svanasana)

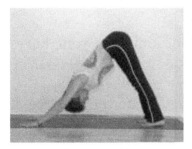

A classical restorative pose, it works towards toning your calves, hamstrings, arms, and belly.

1. From Upward facing dog, exhale and push your hips up so that your body looks like an inverted V.

2. Spread the palms thoroughly and adjust the wrists to stack them under your shoulders.

3. Press your feet towards the mat and push the hips towards the ceiling. If possible, gaze at your thighs.

4. Engage the buttocks and abdomen and hold the posture, breathing deeply, for one minute.

6. Revolved Lunge

From Downward Facing Dog, inhale and lift your leg up and high to the ceiling and place the left foot in between your palms, bending the knee and stacking it over the ankle. Repeat **Revolved Lunge** by **twisting to the left. Hold the posture for one minute.**

7. Chair Pose

Inhale and untwist your Revolve Lunge and sweep your arms over the head and join the palms. *Join the right foot next to the left, bending the knee and pushing your hips back to come into Chair Pose.* Hold for one minute.

To complete the practice, inhale and straighten your knees and torso. Release the hands and relax.

So that was the 7 minute sequence. You can practice it anytime you wish; but just make sure that your tummy is not loaded with food as twisting could upset the digestion otherwise!

Chapter 8: A 30-Minute Daily Routine For Shaping And Toning Your Body

The last sequence, the 7-minute one, is an instant metabolism booster and mood uplifting one. This sequence comprises 14 postures and two Pranayama (breathing) exercises and is meant to help you lose weight, shape, and tone your body and mind.

It is advisable to practice the routine on an empty stomach, preferably in the morning, to reap the maximum out of the practice. However, you can practice at any time, provided your stomach is not packed with food.

So are you ready for the longer, stronger, and more powerful weight loss sequence? Here we go!

30-Minute Yoga for Weight Loss

You can practice this sequence twice to intensify your fat burning potential, but if you are doing it two times back to back, skip the final three steps of the practice after the first round. I will tell you more about those steps at the end of the sequence.

1. Garland Pose/Complete Squat (Malasana)

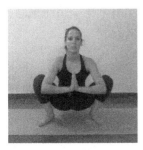

Tone your thighs and hips with this fabulous hip opener. Pay close attention to the way you breathe and how your body reacts while in this posture as it will help you center and ground throughout your practice.

1. Stand straight, legs separated wider than your hips, hands resting on either sides.

2. Exhale and squat completely, feet flat on the mat, and knees open out.

3. Inhale and join the palms at heart center, pushing the knees out with your elbows.

4. Engage the abdominal muscles and pull the navel in towards the spine. Straighten your spine and lean forward slightly without compromising the spine.

5. Press the feet firmly into the mat.

6. Close your eyes, and breathing deeply, hold the posture for 60 seconds.

Tips: *Avoid this posture if you have a knee or ankle injury. You can practice Utkatasana instead.*

2. Standing Forward Fold (Uttanasana)

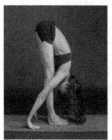 Fold your way forward to improve the circulation to your brain. Relax yourself, boost your digestive ability, and tone your abdomen and hamstrings with this simple posture. Keep your knees bent if you have a back or knee injury.

1. With the final exhalation in Garland pose, place the palms flat on the mat, and stand up. Join the feet together.

2. Exhale and fold forward from your hips, allowing your forehead to rest close to the shin and abdomen on the thighs. If possible, place the palms on either side of the feet.

3. Push your hips back and lengthen the spine. Keep the thighs, buttocks, and abdomen engaged.

4. Close your eyes and hold the posture, breathing deeply, for one minute.

3. Eight-Limbed Salutation/Knees, Chest, and Chin Pose (Ashtanga Namaskara)

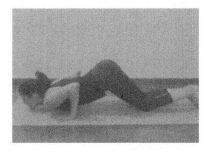

Strengthen and tone your arms while challenging your abdominal muscles with this pose.

1. On an inhale, step your legs back, one at a time, from Uttanasana. Keep the toes tucked.

2. Exhale and place the knees, chest, and chin on the mat. Adjust your position to ensure that the chest rests in between the palms and chin in front.

3. Bring your elbows close to your chest, allowing them to point towards the ceiling.

4. Gaze forward, engage the abdominal muscles, and hold the posture for one minute.

4. Cobra Pose (Bhujangasana)

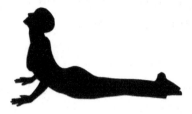

Massage your digestive organs to boost your digestion and tone the abdomen with this gentle backbend. It stretches and tones your back muscles and strengthens your lower back.

1. On an inhale, slither your body forward, stretching the legs back.

2. Pressing the palms firmly into the mat, push your head and chest off the mat, keeping the forearms and elbows on the mat. Your body should be off the mat only till your navel.

3. Keep stretching back until you feel a tingle on your lower back. Keep the buttocks and core muscles engaged.

4. Gaze forward and breathing deeply, hold the posture for a minute.

5. Bow Pose (Dhanurasana)

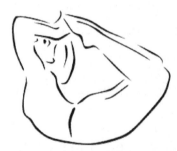

This posture works on your entire body and tones it. It also improves your metabolism and digestion, two important factors for weight loss.

1. With the last exhalation in Cobra Pose, lie down on the mat.

2. Bend the legs at knee and bring your feet close to the buttocks.

3. Hold your ankles with respective hands.

4. Inhale and lift your head and chest off the mat until you are balancing on your navel. Exhale and pull your legs away from your body so that your thighs and knees are also off the mat. Tilt your head back and gaze up.

5. Breathing deeply, hold the posture for one minute.

6. Child's Pose (Balasana)

 This is a restorative pose that will give you a break during the practice, at the same time working towards toning your thighs. This pose is a variation of the classical Child's pose.

1. With the last exhalation in Dhanurasana, release the legs and rest the palms at chest level.

2. Pushing the palms into the mat, take a deep breath, and push yourself to lift your torso and come on your knees.

3. Exhale and sit back on your heels, separating the knees wider than your hips. Stretch your hands to the front and let the forehead rest on the mat. Allow your abdomen to rest in between your thighs.

4. Breathe deeply into the posture and hold it for a minute.

7. Boat Pose (Navasana/Naukasana)

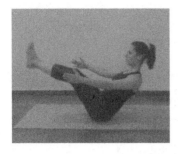

If I had to choose just one pose to tone the entire body, then my choice would be the Boat Pose. A great core sculptor, it helps to strengthen your back while shaping your arms and legs.

1. From Balasana, inhale and straighten your torso and stretch the legs out to the front. Lengthen your spine.

2. On an exhale, stretch and lift your legs and torso from the mat, keeping the abdominal muscles engaged. Slightly lean backwards to balance your body on your sitting bones. Stretch out your arms so that they are parallel to the mat.

3. In the final posture, your body and legs should make an angle of 45 degrees. Feel free to keep the knees bent if you have back or knee injuries.

4. Hold the posture for one minute, breathing deeply into the posture.

Tips: *You can keep the fingertips on the mat till your core becomes stronger.*

8. Upward Plank Pose (Purvottanasana)

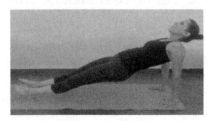

This is a counter pose for Boat Pose. In addition, it is a overall body stretching and sculpting posture.

1. With the final exhalation in Boat Pose, release the legs and place the palms just behind your buttocks with fingertips facing you.

2. On an inhale, press the palms and lift your torso off the mat, head tilting back.

3. Keep the legs stretched out, extending the toes forward.

4. Tuck the chin slightly and, keeping the abdomen and buttocks engaged, hold the posture for a minute.

Tip: If you have a back or knee injury, bend your knees, keeping the feet flat on the mat, and separate your knees and feet as wide as your hips.

9. Seated Forward Fold (Paschimottanasana)

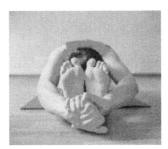

The forward bend enhances the power of your digestive organs and tones the abdominal region. It also elongates the spine and massages the back.

1. On the last exhale in Purvottanasana, place your torso back on the mat.

2. Ensure that sitting bones are resting on the mat.

3. Flex your feet towards you.

4. Inhale and swing the arms over your head. Exhale and forward fold from the hips, resting the abdomen on the thighs. If possible, hold your feet from outside. Alternatively,

you can place your palms on your shin or on either side of your leg. Let your forehead rest on your shin.

5. Take a short breath in and as you breathe out, deepen your bend a little more.

6. Hold the posture, breathing deeply, for a minute.

Tip: Keep the knees bent if you have a back or knee injury. The idea is to lengthen the spine and hence, you can keep the knee bent to hold your feet.

10. Seated Spinal Twist (Ardha Matsyendrasana)

Twists are detoxifiers and this one is no exception. Bonus – you will be awarded with a toned abdomen and back.

How to do it:

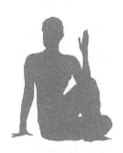

1. On an inhale, straighten your torso.

2. Bend your right knee and place your right sole close to left sitting bones.

3. Cross your left leg over the right, placing one knee over the other.

4. Place your left palm on your back, fingertips pointing away from you.

5. Inhale and lift your right hand. On an exhale, bring your right elbow outside the left knee and try to hold the left ankle. Simultaneously, twist to your left and look over your left shoulder.

6. Hold the posture for a minute.

7. Inhale and release the posture.

8. Repeat on other side for one minute.

11. Bridge Pose (Setu Bhanda Sarvangasana)

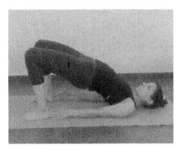

It is an inversion-cum backbend that helps to strengthen your legs and hips. Therapeutic for thyroid and uterus issues, it tones your back and abdomen.

1. Straighten both legs out after you complete the previous posture and lie down on your back.

2. Bend the knees and separate them at hip distance, planting the feet firmly into the mat. Bring the heels slightly closer to your buttocks. Let the arms rest on either side of the body, palms facing the mat.

3. Inhale, lift your hips, lower and upper back off the mat. (Follow this order when you lift your body)

4. Engage the buttocks and core, tuck your chin to the chest, and keep lifting the hip up.

5. If possible, hold your ankles with respective hands.

6. Breathing deeply, hold the posture for a minute.

12. Wind Relieving Pose (Pavanamuktasana)

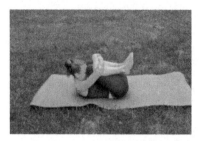

End the bloating and boost your digestion with this tummy toning yoga posture. It also massages your back and relieves tension.

1. With the final exhalation in Bridge pose, release your body gently on the mat.

2. Hug your knees to the chest and bind them using your arms.

3. On an inhale, press the thighs into the abdomen while lifting the head and chest so that head and knee touch each other.

4. Exhale and hold the posture for about a minute.

Tip: Keep the head and chest on the mat if you have shoulder injuries.

13. Reclining Abdominal Twist (Supta Vakrasana)

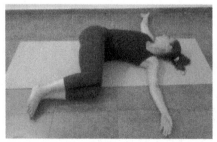

This twist massages your spine while helping you get rid of toxins. It promotes digestion through its block and release mechanism.

1. On an exhale, release the head and chest to the mat, without changing the knees. Stretch out the hands at shoulder level.

2. Inhale and as you exhale, place your knees to the right and twist your torso to the left. Look to your left. Focus on lifting the knee close to the chest while pushing the left shoulder on the mat.

3. Hold the posture for a minute.

4. Inhale and come back to the center.

5. Exhale and repeat on the other side.

14. Corpse Pose (Shavasana)

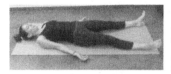 Relax your body, allowing yourself to let go with this classical restorative pose.

1. On an inhale, come back to the center. Exhale and stretch out the legs wider than your hips, allowing the feet to fall away naturally.

2. Keep the arms away from the body, allowing space for armpits to breathe. Curl the fingers naturally.

3. Tuck the chin slightly towards the chest to make space for your neck.

4. Relax the entire body, close your eyes, and lie down in Corpse pose for 5 minutes.

15. Bellows Breathing - Bhastrika Pranayama

It is a powerful way to eliminate toxins, boost your metabolism, and tone your abdomen. Since the breathing technique involves powerful and rapid inhalations and exhalations, it is advisable to refrain from this practice if you have hypertension or heart issues or if you are menstruating.

1. Sit down in a comfortable seated posture where your spine will be erect for the next 5-minute practice.

2. Take 5 rounds of deep inhalations and exhalations to prepare your body for the practice.

3. Inhale and exhale powerfully and rapidly through your nose, producing a hissing sound in the process. As you exhale, allow the abdomen to fall into the rib cavity close to your spine.

4. Do this for 1 minute. Follow up with three rounds of normal breathing and resume the Bhastrika practice.

5. Continue practicing the same way for 5 minutes.

16. Anulom Vilom Pranayama (Alternate Nostril Breathing)

It is a calming and restorative breath that helps you to let go of stress. Stress is said to be one of the major culprits behind belly fat. So eliminating this factor would help in weight loss and toning.

1. Sit down in any comfortable seated posture, keeping your spine erect and aligned with neck and head.

2. Rest your palms on your knees.

3. Let the thumb and index finger of left hand be in touch while the other three fingers are extended out.

4. Lift your right arm at chest level. Place the middle and index finger in between your eyebrows. Use the right thumb to close your right nostril and the right ring finger to close your left nostril. Extend the little finger to the ceiling.

5. Close your eyes. Close the right nostril and exhale completely through your left nostril.

6. Take a slow, deep inhalation through the left nostril for a count of 4. Close the left nostril, open the right nostril, and exhale for a count of 8.

7. Now, inhale through the right for a count of 4, close the right, open the left, and exhale for a count of 8.

This completes one round of Anulom Vilom Pranayama. Continue practicing for 5 minutes more.

Once you complete the breathing practice, breathe normally. Rub your palms to generate heat. Place them on your eyes; open your eyes and look into your palms. Join the palms and bow to Mother Earth for the lovely support she gave you during the practice.

What if you want to practice longer? It is advisable to stretch your practice to 60 minutes to get more out of the practice. If you're planning to do so, practice only 'till ***Pose 13 (reclining abdominal twist). From there proceed to Pose 1 or Garland Pose in the following way.***

1. Once you complete Reclining abdominal twist on either side, roll to your right and sit upright.

2. Bend your knees, placing the feet firmly on the mat. Separate the knees as wide as your hips and squat and come into Garland pose.

Repeat the entire sequence once more before resting in Shavasana and continuing with the breathing practice.

For those who love chanting, you can chant this Shanti Mantra as you bow forward:

"Om Saha Nau-Avatu

Saha Nau Bhunaktu

Saha Viiryam Karavaavahai

Tejasvi Nau-Adhiitam-Astu Maa Vidvissaavahai

Om Shaantih Shaantih Shaantihi"

This is what it means!

May god protect us both (the teacher and the student),

May God nourish us both,

May we work together with energy and vigor,

May our study be enlightening and not give rise to hostility,

Om, peace, peace, peace.

So when are you going to start your yoga practice to shed that excess flab from your mind and body?

Chapter 9: 15 Minutes A Day For A Stress-Free Life

Stress is irritating; it just eats up your life, leaving nothing, but frustration and tiredness. But now you can use the power of your breath to relax your body and mind by practicing just 15 minutes every day.

The sequence comprises just 6 yoga poses along with one of the most effective stress busting breathing techniques – abdominal breathing. All the postures are restorative in nature, helping you relax and unwind. Feel free to hold the poses longer, 5 minutes or more, if you wish to go really deep into each one of them.

A 15-Minute Fix for Stress

1. Reclining Bound Angle (Supta Baddha Konasana)

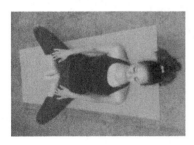 It is a heart and hip opener that helps you release all the pent-up emotions from these two areas.

1. Sit on the floor, bend the knees and join the soles of your feet.

2. Place your palms on either side of your knees.

3. Place a bolster at the end of your spine and start reclining, bending the elbows and supporting your torso.

4. Once your back is completely on the bolster, rest the hands on either side of your chest, palms facing up and fingers facing back.

5. Close your eyes and relax.

6. Hold the posture, breathing deeply, for 5 minutes. As you inhale, let your abdomen rise. With each exhalation, allow the stomach to fall close to the spine.

7. To come out, press the elbows onto the floor and come back to starting position.

Tip: Place two blocks under your knees to support them if you are unable to get your knees on the floor.

2. Simple Seated Twist (Bharadvajasana)

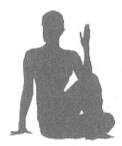 There are many variations of this posture. So you choose a posture that suits you best. If you have knee injuries, you can join the soles of your feet to sit in Baddha Konasana and twist. The pose I have mentioned here is Bharadvajasana.

1. Once you come back to seated posture from the previous pose, stretch out the legs. Bend the knees and rest your buttocks on the heels.

2. Inhale and shift the buttocks to your left and knees to the right.

3. Place your right palm under the left thigh. Swing your left hand behind you and hold the crease of your right elbow.

4. Exhale and twist to your left. Hold the posture for one minute, by breathing into your abdomen.

5. Inhale and come back to kneeling.

6. Repeat on the other side.

Tips: If your are sitting in Sukhasana or Baddha Konasana, place your right palm on the left knee, hold the right elbow crease with your left hand and twist to the left. Repeat the same on the other side.

3. Seated Bound Angle (Baddha Konasana)

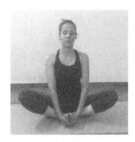
It is the seated version of the posture with which you started your practice. Hips is where we generally store stress and hence, practicing the hip openers will help you calm down and relax.

1. Stretch out the legs after your complete the twist.

2. Bend the knees and join the soles of your feet. Keep your feet at a comfortable distance from your pelvis where you will still feel the stretch on your groins and hips.

3. Place your palms on your knees, pushing them closer to the floor.

4. Inhale and straighten your spine.

5. Exhale and bend forward so that your navel comes close to the spine. Keep pushing the knees close to the floor.

6. Hold the posture while practicing abdominal breathing for one minute.

Tips: Place a cushion or bolster to ensure that the sitting bones are on the mat.

4. Seated Wide Angle Pose (Upavishta Konasana)

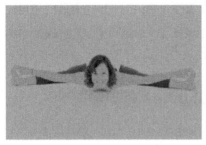

Along with helping you let go of everything that doesn't serve you, this yoga posture eases digestive issues and tones your thighs. It heals your back ache and lengthens your spine.

1. From Baddha Konasana, straighten your torso and extend your legs as wide as possible, keeping your knees straight. Flex the toes towards you.

2. Inhale, lift your arms over your head and lengthen your spine.

3. Exhale and fold forward from your hips, holding the big toe with a three-finger grip. [Three finger grip – hold the big toe using the thumb, index, and middle fingers of respective hands in such a way that the thumb rests on top of your big toe.]

4. Fold forward as much as possible without rounding your spine. If possible let your chest and chin rest on the floor.

5. Hold the posture for one minute, breathing in and out of your abdomen.

Tips: Keep your knee slightly bent if you have knee, ligament, or back injuries. Choose to sit on folded blankets or cushion to keep your sitting bones flat on the floor.

5. Happy Baby Pose (Ananda Balasana)

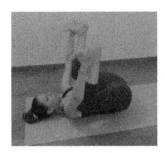

Babies are always happy and hence, the pose gets its name from the way they just hold their toes, smiling, showing their happiness. This pose, as with previous postures, focuses on opening up your hips and releasing the unwanted emotions stored there.

1. Inhale and slowly straighten your torso from the previous pose. Join your legs and lie down on your back.

2. Inhale and lift your leg up, keeping the knees bent, and hold the big toe using the three-finger grip. Let the feet face the ceiling as you pull the knees as close to the floor as possible.

3. Keep the hips and lower back on the floor.

4. Hold the posture, practicing abdominal breathing, for one minute.

6. Crocodile Pose (Makarasana)

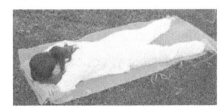

This is a restorative posture; not that popular as the Corpse Pose but highly effective in helping you relax.

1. Release your feet on the mat and stretch out your legs from Happy Baby pose.

2. Roll on to lie down on your stomach.

3. Make a pillow by placing your arms atop each other and rest the forehead on it.

4. Separate the legs slightly wider than your hips and allow them to rest naturally.

5. Close your eyes and breathing deeply, hold the posture for 5 minutes.

When you are ready to wind up the practice, gently move your toes and fingers. Remove the pillow from your forehead and move your head from side to side. Roll to your right, and sit in any seated posture of your choice. Keep your eyes closed. Rub your palm to generate heat and place it over your eyes.

Take a deep breath in and exhale completely. Join your palms at heart center and extend a word of gratitude to your Higher Self for such a wonderful practice.

As I mentioned earlier, you can hold each of the poses for 5 or more minutes, allowing your body to become more and more relaxed. Feel free to use any props you might need to feel completely relaxed.

You might see changes with a single practice session, but to keep the benefits with you for a longer period, practice daily!

Chapter 10: Mudras For Weight Loss

Mudra is a Sanskrit word that means gestures. In yogic terms, mudras refer to the way we hold our body or shape our fingers so as to channelize the flow of energy. This chapter refers to five hand mudras you can use as a supplementary aid with your yoga and meditation practice.

5 Mudras That Help in Weight Loss

1. Surya Mudra

Our body, according to ancient science, is made up of five natural elements – air, water, fire, earth, and ether. An inactive fire leads to fat deposits. This particular mudra focuses on stimulating and enhancing this fire, boosting fat metabolism. At the same time, it restores the natural levels of the Earth element.

1. Sit down in a comfortable seated posture keeping your eyes closed and relaxing your body.

2. Rest your palms on your knees, palms facing up.

3. Rest the tip of the ring finger on the base of the thumb, pressing the thumb gently on the top of the ring finger.

[This positioning helps to suppress the Earth element while triggering the Fire.]

Practice for 15 to 30 minutes.

2. Linga Mudra

Linga means phallus. This mudra also works towards improving your metabolism, the key to burning off excess fat.

1. Sit down in Baddha Konasana. Keep cushions or blocks under your knees for support, if your knees are not on the floor.

2. Interlock your palms in front of your body at the level of your navel and extend your left thumb towards the ceiling.

3. Close your eyes and meditate.

You can practice this whenever you want, but ideally, it is advisable to practice it thrice a day for 15 minutes each.

3. Apan Mudra

Good digestion is the key to weight loss. Give your digestion, and thus your metabolism, the much wanted boost with this Mudra. It promotes detoxification as well as digestion.

1. Sit in any comfortable seated posture. Relax your body and close your eyes.
2. Let your palms rest on your knees, palms facing up.
3. Join the tips of thumb, middle, and ring fingers, stretching out the little and the index finger.
4. Practice with both hands for 45 minutes.

If you are unable to practice for 45 minutes in one go, aim for splitting it into three sessions of 15 minutes each.

4. Vyan Mudra

Stress is a major culprit behind unwanted weight gain. Now put your cortisol to rest and bring your swaggering blood pressure under control with this Mudra.

1. Sit down in a comfortable seated posture. Close your eyes and relax your body, keeping the spine erect.

2. Rest your palms on the knees, palms facing up.

3. Join the tips of thumb, middle, and index fingers. Stretch out your ring and little finger.

Practice it for 15 to 20 minutes every day, thrice a day.

5. Shunya Mudra

Shunya means emptiness and this one does wonders by regulating your thyroid, bringing in weight loss.

1. Sit down in a comfortable seated posture. Close your eyes and relax your body, keeping the spine erect.

2. Rest your palms on the knees, palms facing up.

3. Rest the tips of middle fingers on the base of the respective thumbs, pressing the thumbs on the middle finger.

4. Stretch out the other fingers.

Practice for 20 to 30 minutes daily.

Make sure that you practice these mudras daily and consistently, even if you have to skip your yoga practice due to some reason. One of the best things I love about the mudras is that it gives you the flexibility to practice anywhere. Put on your headphones and listen to some binaural beats that would help you meditate without losing focus.

Chapter 11: Visualization For Weight Loss

Creative visualization, while meditating, has been hailed by many as a powerful tool for shedding excess weight. Using this technique, you convince your subconscious mind to shape the body you wish to create, thus making use of the body-mind connection.

With regular efforts, the subconscious mind accepts that this new body image of yours is real, with your body eventually working towards making this mental image come true. You can also use visualization to reduce the quantity of food you eat, follow a healthy diet, and exercise regularly, slowly coaxing yourself to achieve your goal.

Here is a small visualization practice that you could do after your yoga practice to boost the results of your weight loss yoga regimen.

15 Minute Visualization for Shedding the Excess Pounds

1. Sit down in a comfortable seated posture. Let your palms rest on your knees. Close your eyes and take a few deep breaths to consciously relax your body. Just observe your breath. If you mind wanders away, bring it gently to concentrate on your breath.

2. Once you are ready, start visualizing a stream of white light flowing into your body from a powerfully infinite source.

Do not try to find or create a source. Just experience the beautiful light flood into each and every cell of your body.

3. **Imagine a powerful beam of white light**, all the way through your scalp, penetrating into your body.

4. **Allow the healing light to flow into each and every cell of your body, taking away all the unwanted fat and toxins with it.** Do not resist or judge whatever is happening; just enjoy and allow the detoxification and cleansing to take place.

5. When you feel that you are completely cleansed, **imagine a whirlpool opening up from your navel. Now, allow the whirlpool to suck in the white light, along with the fat and toxins it has absorbed.**

6. As the white light disappears, feel your body becoming light and toned. Keep repeating this affirmation – "It is easy for me to lose weight. I now have a healthy body and mind. I radiate happiness and vitality."

7. Once you feel you are ready, open your eyes and step into the world with renewed energy and spirits.

Just trust that you have already achieved your goal. Relax and let go of anything and everything that does not serve you.

Listen to your body and you will find that losing weight is quite simple!

Chapter 12: Finding The Perfect Yoga Studio

So, now that you've got all the stuff you need, there's only thing to do. Find the perfect place. While many people just follow the good old "try and you'll see" technique, there are a few strategies you can use which might prove helpful.

Seeing that so many people swear by it, why not try out different studios before you make up your mind? There are probably introductory classes, and there's no obligation to commit to anything during it. Explain that you're just trying it out and we're sure that there won't be any problems. This will allow you to see firsthand if this studio and this instructor are right for you.

In addition, try observing the people around you during this first class. Are they the kind of yoga community you're looking for? Do you see yourself here a couple of times a week, with these exact people?

Similarly, we can't forget the location. Try finding something that's close to you, or convenient, seeing that something that's inconvenient isn't likely to become a part of your routine. The same goes for the price: you should be happy to pay for what you're getting and not feel like you're being ripped off. Sometimes, the most expensive yoga studios aren't really the best ones. They might be more frequented, but again, pay attention to the people who go there. Are they your kind of people?

Furthermore, make sure that the yoga studio of your choice has a wide variety of choices. You might want to switch to a different yoga class at one point and it'd be more convenient to do it within the same yoga studio, instead of looking for a new one every time.

Likewise, make sure you like the instructor. This is one of the most important things. A good instructor continues learning at every stage. A good instructor not only teaches you, but challenges you, pushes you beyond what you thought possible. They inspire you not only with their words, but with their actions. So, for a full blown impact, choose this kind of a person for the privilege of being your yoga instructor.

Chapter 13: 5 Things Every Beginner Should Know About Yoga

1. Practice makes perfect

As it was previously mentioned, yoga is for everyone who isn't looking for a miracle cure, but rather who is willing to invest time and effort into creating a better life quality for himself/herself and those around them. Anything that is worth doing is done and achieved through sweat and hard work. Yoga is one of those things. But, luckily for you, it offers a lot of positive side-effects, too. If you can't do something right from the first try, don't give up. Always keep trying and eventually, you are bound to do it.

2. Intricate, pretzel-like poses don't make an expert

Yes, we all agree that it looks absolutely mind-numbing seeing a yoga expert twist himself into all sorts of knots and pretzels. But, that's not the point of yoga. Every single body is flexible to its own extent, and we shouldn't push our own body over the boundaries it is not yet ready to go. Yoga is all about a peace of mind and spiritual unity, which in all honesty, can be achieved in any pose, pretzel or not. So, you be proud while you do your Mountain or your Tree pose, and know that it doesn't matter who can bend and twist the most. It's not a competition, it is a state of mind.

3. Don't compare yourself to others

You might succumb to doing this, especially in the beginning and especially when you see advanced yoga practitioners in your class. Why would you do this to yourself? Have you forgotten that all those experts were once beginners, too, just like you are now? They practiced hard to reach this level, which means that you can reach it, too. It's all a question of character, desire and perseverance.

4. Watch your breathing

It's essential that you watch your breathing during your yoga workouts. You should always have a steady flow of breath, to achieve maximum awareness. If you find yourself out of breath or making short, violent breaths, better take a break. Don't push it, because you are not really relaxing your body, you are pushing it. Take a break and then continue, being mindful of your breathing.

5. Never skip Savasana

Savasana is very simple: you basically just lie down at the end of class. Due to its seeming triviality, many people think it carries no weight and are all too eager to skip it. Don't be one of those people! It's very important, because it allows your body as well as your mind to relax and unwind, and to store the value of the poses you just did for long-term usage. Yoga should never end abruptly, which is true of almost every physical activity. You should always ease out of it, and Savasana offers you the perfect way to do so.

6. Don't forget to enjoy!

Last, but definitely not least is to remember to always enjoy yourself. If you try yoga and you don't like how it makes you feel, take a break. Maybe you will change your mind later. Whatever it is that you like and enjoy doing, yoga should always complement it, never be in contrast with it. So, remember to open your heart and mind, and strive to reach for spiritual peace of mind and body!

Chapter 14: Additional Tips

OK, so you know what to do now, but we thought we might paint a few more pictures here. For example, imagine yourself at a yoga class. Everything is super Zen, relaxed, everyone is in a state of perfect bliss. Then, all of a sudden, you hear a familiar ring tone! Oh my gosh! Did you forget to turn off your phone? Yup. You certainly did. But, don't worry, it happens to everyone. One of the things you can do to avoid this is leave your cell at home. After all, you're going there to zone out of everything. Why would you need your phone then?

Also, make sure to wear form fitting clothes, seeing you'll be doing a lot of bending, so you don't really want any strangers (be they guys or gals) looking down your loose t-shirt. The same goes for leggings. Before you buy them, make sure they're not see through, as this sometimes happens.

If you choose a popular yoga studio, get ready for a sardine party. It's quite possible that there will be so many of you that your mat will be right next to someone else's giving you very little personal space. Still, small though it may be, it's yours and as such, precious. The same goes for other people. Make sure you don't impose on their personal space and make sure not to fall on anyone. Can you imagine the domino effect it would cause?

Conclusion

Thank you again for buying this book!

I hope it was able to help you find out what yoga is all about.

The next step is to find the perfect yoga studio and start achieving that peace of mind everyone is talking about!

Oh! And one more thing...

...I Need Your Help!

I honestly hope that you enjoyed my book as much as I enjoyed writing it.

It is my goal to make this read enjoyable and worthy of your money as we, together, discover the world of Yoga in this introduction book for beginners.

It would mean the world to me if you spent 5 minutes of your (precious, trust me, I know!) time to leave a review for me on Amazon. You would do a person a huge HUGE favor and you would help me a lot with my goal to keep writing books that will make this world a better place.I read all the reviews, I respect every single one of them and I appreciate whatever you have to say about it, good or bad!

I wouldn't be able to thank you enough if you did this favor for me... may good energy follow you everywhere you go! :D

Thank you and I wholeheartedly wish you the very best in your life!

Namaste ☺

Made in the USA
Las Vegas, NV
31 March 2021

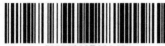